My Skinny Lil' Diet

How to lose up to 30lbs
In
30 Days

By
New York Times Best Selling Author
Carmen Bryan

My Skinny Lil' Diet

By
New York Times Best Selling Author
Carmen Bryan

DIET AND MEAL PLAN
DISCLAIMER

The information provided in My Skinny Lil Diet is designed for informational purposes only. Before beginning this or any diet and or meal plan it is your sole responsibility to seek advice from your physician.

All information provided including the meal plan is not individualized and is not intended to be a substitute for professional medical advice.

Part One

Transform your life in one month.

You're just a step away from losing the weight. "My Skinny Lil' Diet" is a seven hundred and fifty calorie a day diet that is uniquely designed to help you drop the weight quickly, safely and naturally.

All suggested meals are packed with nutrient rich foods including lean meats, fish and fresh fruits and vegetables.

Our goal is to make life a little easier by providing daily meal plans with alternatives for the next thirty days as you embark on this life changing journey.

Part Two
Getting Started

The hardest part of any diet is getting started. Most often we let our fears and past failures break our will and determine our fate. Now that you've made the decision to lose the weight, you can begin your journey with confidence.

The next step requires you to clear out your cabinets and refrigerator. Get rid of anything that is not in the glossary and that will tempt you to stray from the meal plans. Distractions have a tendency to create unnecessary obstacles.

Your next order of business will be to create a shopping list from the variety of fresh meats, fish, poultry, fruits and vegetables from the glossary.

You have the option to substitute foods from the glossary as long as the daily calories amount to seven hundred and fifty.

It is also recommended that you drink plenty of water daily and refrain from strenuous physical exercise and aerobics on this meal program. If at any time during this diet or any diet you begin to feel ill, nauseous or faint, eat something immediately and contact a physician or visit your local emergency room.

Part Three
THE JOURNEY
Day 1

Nothing holds more power over the body than the mind. Your thoughts have the ability to influence the physical and bring about what you desire. Envision the perfect you and take a mental picture. Every day for the next thirty days, visualize the new you and repeat out loud 'I'm losing weight with no difficulty.' Now is the time to reprogram the mind. Think thin!

BREAKFAST

1 cup of black coffee or tea	1 calorie
1 tangerine	47 calories
½ bagel	122 calories

LUNCH

3.5 ounces of lean chicken breast	140 calories
1 cup of raw or steamed broccoli	50 calories
1 cup of raspberries	65 calories

DINNER

3.5 ounces of lean beef	200 calories
1 cup of asparagus	32 calories
1 cup of steamed carrots	53 calories
1 breadsticks	12 calories
1 plum	30 calories

Day 2

It's day two, a new dawn a new day and a day where anything is possible. Today is the perfect day to take charge of your thoughts. If you are having negatives thoughts, think of something different. With a new image comes a new frame of mind and new way of life.

BREAKFAST

1 cup of black coffee or tea	1 calorie
½ banana	52 calories

LUNCH

3.5 ounces of lean veal	200 calories
1 cup of green cabbage	25 calories
½ slice of wheat bread	39 calories
½ cup of blueberries	41 calories
1 plum	30 calories

DINNER

1 pound of shrimp	200 calories
1 cup of string beans	44 calories
1 cup of steamed Carrots	53 calories
1 breadstick	12 calories
1 pear	51 calories

Day 3

Change is inevitable and very necessary. If you are not happy with your current weight, then change it. Change your thoughts and you will change your life.

BREAKFAST

1 cup of black coffee or tea	1 calorie
1 nectarine	50 calories
1 bread stick	12 calories

LUNCH

2 lobsters tails	160 calories
2 cups of spinach	48 calories
1 cup of beets	8 calories
2 breadsticks	24 calories
1 cup of strawberries	46 calories

DINNER

3.5 ounces of filleted fish	160 calories
1 cup of romaine lettuce	30 calories
1 cup of tomatoes	35 calories
1 cup of broccoli	50 calories
½ slice of wheat bread	39 calories
1 cup of watermelon	85 calories

Day 4

We all have had thoughts of changing the world, but the true challenge is changing within. The ability to change conquers all other abilities.

BREAKFAST

1 cup of black coffee or tea	1 calorie
1 peach	59 calories
1 breadstick	12 calories

LUNCH

1 pound of crab legs	200 calories
1 cup of string beans	44 calories
1 cup of cucumbers	14 calories
1 plum	30 calories
1 breadstick	12 calories

DINNER

3 ounces of lean lamb chops	250 calories
1 cup of shredded bok choy	10 calories
1 cup of kale	42 calories
½ slice of wheat bread	39 calories
1 kiwi	40 calories

Day 5

Anything you create, you can recreate.
Concentrate on the out-come, the perfect you and
allow the powers within to assist you on your
path. Dwell only on the positive.

BREAKFAST

1 cup of black coffee or tea	1 calorie
1 pear	51 calories
½ bagel	122 calories

LUNCH

4 ounces turkey chops	120 calories
1 cup of zucchini	33 calories
½ cup of white potatoes	81 calories
1 cup of beets	8 calories
1 breadstick	12 calories
1 peach	59 calories

DINNER

3.5 ounces of lean chicken breast	140 calories
1 cup of romaine lettuce	30 calories
1 cup of tomatoes	35 calories
1 breadstick	12 calories
1 cup of strawberries	46 calories

Day 6

It is day six and you're doing great. Remember thoughts become things. Focus only on what you want to appear in your life. We are what we think about.

BREAKFAST

1 cup of black coffee or tea	1 calorie
½ banana	52 calories
1 breadstick	12 calories

LUNCH

3.5 ounces of lean beef	200 calories
1 cup of chicory greens	42 calories
½ cup of corn	45 calories
1 breadstick	12 calories
½ cup of blueberries	41 calories

DINNER

3.5 ounces of lean veal	200 calories
1 cup of broccoli	50 calories
1 cup of tomatoes	35 calories
1 Melba toast	12 calories
½ cup of grapes	51 calories

Day 7

Don't forget to love yourself today. The key to happiness is self-love. Regardless of your weight, you are a beautiful and magnificent being. Congratulate yourself for getting through the first week, you deserve it!

BREAKFAST

1 cup of black coffee or tea	1 calorie
1 grape fruit	37 calories
½ slice of wheat bread	39 calories

LUNCH

1 pound of shrimp	200 calories
1 cup of snow peas	26 calories
½ cup of carrots	26 calories
1 Melba toast	12 calories
1 pomegranate	72 calories

DINNER

3.5 ounces of lean beef	200 calories
1 cup of asparagus	32 calories
½ cup of fresh corn	45 calories
1 breadstick	12 calories
½ cup of cherries	51 calories

Day 8

Challenges help develop strength. There is no doubt that this is a difficult journey, however there is also no doubt that you will make it to the end. Stay focused and keep your eyes on the prize.

BREAKFAST

1 cup of black coffee or tea	1 calorie
½ cup of honey dew melon	50 calories
1 breadstick	14 calories

LUNCH

1 pound of crab legs	200 calories
1 cup of broccoli	50 calories
½ cup of potatoes	81 calories
½ slice of wheat bread	39 calories
1 orange	65 calories

DINNER

3.5 ounces of lean turkey breast	140 calories
1 cup of string beans	44 calories
1 cup of beets	8 calories
1 breadstick	12 calories
1 cup of raspberries	46 calories

Day 9

Thoughts are mere moments just waiting to happen. Keep them pure and active. Doing nothing creates nothing. Take action today by keeping the faith and believing in the new you.

BREAKFAST

1 cup of black coffee or tea	1 calorie
1 plum	30 calories
½ bagel	122 calories

LUNCH

3.5 ounces of filleted fish	160 calories
1 cup of spinach	12 calories
1 cup of carrots	53 calories
½ cup of grapes	32 calories
½ slice of wheat bread	39 calories

DINNER

3.5 ounces of lean beef	200 calories
1 cup of cucumbers	14 calories
1 cup of mushrooms	21 calories
1 breadstick	12 calories
1 pear	51 calories

Day 10

Sometimes when we have our hearts set on something, out of habit we tend to contemplate the worst and give up before reaching the finish line. Break old bad habits and focus on all the unending possibilities that life has to offer.

BREAKFAST

1 cup of black coffee or tea	1 calorie
1 nectarine	59 calories
½ bagel	122 calories

LUNCH

3 ounces of lean lamb chops	250 calories
1 cup of cabbage	25 calories
½ cup of strawberries	23 calories

DINNER

4 ounces of fresh scallops	128 calories
1 cup of string beans	44 calories
1 cup of steamed Carrots	53 calories
1 breadstick	12 calories
½ cup of cherries	37 calories

Day 11

The mind can be your greatest enemy or your greatest ally. All you need to lose weight is you. Let your hearts' desire be the driving force that keeps you focused on your diet and goals. The greater the goal, the greater the reward.

BREAKFAST

1 cup of black coffee or tea	1 calorie
1 pear	51 calories
½ slice of wheat bread	39 calories

LUNCH

2 lobsters tails	160 calories
1 cup of asparagus	32 calories
1 Melba toast	12 calories
1 apple	81 calories

DINNER

3.5 ounces of lean beef	200 calories
1 cup of string beans	44 calories
1 cup of carrots	53 calories
2 breadsticks	24 calories
1 kiwi	40 calories

Day 12

Experience the new you through faith, determination and discipline. Sticking to the plan will lead to many benefits that will ultimately change your life for the better. Let nothing distract you from your goal.

BREAKFAST

1 cup of black coffee or tea	1 calorie
½ cup of blueberries	50 calories
1 breadstick	12 calories

LUNCH

3.5 ounces of lean chicken breast	160 calories
1 cup of shredded Bok Choy	20 calories
1 cup of snow peas	26 calories
½ slice of wheat bread	39 calories
1 nectarine	59 calories

DINNER

1 pound of crab legs	200 calories
2 cups of broccoli	100 calories
½ cup of carrots	26 calories
1 peach	59 calories

Day 13

With change comes struggle and with struggle comes progress. Progress always leads to happiness.

BREAKFAST

1 cup of black coffee or tea	1 calorie
½ cup of strawberries	23 calories
½ banana	52 calories
1 breadstick	12 calories

LUNCH

3.5 ounces of lean turkey breast	140 calories
1 cup of snow peas	26 calories
1 cup of mushrooms	21 calories
½ slice of wheat bread	39 calories
1 plum	30 calories

DINNER

3 ounces of lean lamb chops	250 calories
1 cup of broccoli	50 calories
1 cup of mushrooms	21 calories
1 cup of spinach	24 calories
1 breadstick	12 calories
1 pear	51 calories

Day 14

Congratulations! You made it to week two. There is nothing you can't accomplish when you put your mind to it. Just keep doing the things you need to do in order to create a new you.

BREAKFAST

1 cup of black coffee or tea	1 calorie
1 cup of grapes	62 calories
1 slice of wheat bread	78 calories

LUNCH

3.5 ounces of lean veal	200 calories
1 cup of romaine lettuce	30 calories
1 cup of tomatoes	35 calories
1 breadstick	12 calories
½ cup of blueberries	41 calories
1 plum	30 calories

DINNER

4 ounces of lean turkey chops	120 calories
1 cup of spinach	24 calories
1 cup of steamed Carrots	53 calories
1 breadstick	12 calories
1 pear	51 calories

Day 15

You are half way there. Take some time to reward yourself with something special for all the hard work you have put in over these last two weeks. Stay focused and stay strong, you are almost there.

BREAKFAST

1 cup of black coffee or tea	1 calorie
1 nectarine	59 calories
2 breadsticks	24 calories

LUNCH

1 pound of crab legs	200 calories
1 cup of red cabbage	20 calories
1 cup of zucchini	33 calories
1 Melba toast	12 calories
½ cup of blueberries	41 calories

DINNER

3.5 ounces of lean beef	200 calories
1 cup of zucchini	33 calories
1 cup of tomatoes	35 calories
1 cup of beets	8 calories
1 breadstick	12 calories
½ cup of strawberries	51 calories

Day 16

Within you is the ability to create and transform. Knowing who you are is essential to your progress. Believe in yourself today and discover your true power.

BREAKFAST

1 cup of black coffee or tea	1 calorie
1 plum	30 calories
½ bagel	122 calories

LUNCH

1 pound of shrimp	200 calories
½ cup of potatoes	81 calories
1 Melba toast	12 calories
½ cup of honeydew	24 calories

DINNER

3.5 ounces of lean chicken breast	140 calories
1 cup of eggplant	20 calories
½ cup of swiss chard	3 calories
2 breadsticks	24 calories
1 cup of watermelon	85 calories

Day 17

You are beautiful just as you are. Losing the weight will only enhance your beauty-not create it. When you feel good, you look good. Today, celebrate the natural beauty in you.

BREAKFAST

1 cup of black coffee or tea	1 calorie
½ cup of strawberries	23 calories
½ bagel	122 calories

LUNCH

3.5 ounces of lean veal	200 calories
1 cup of green cabbage	25 calories
½ slice of wheat bread	39 calories
½ cup of blueberries	41 calories

DINNER

2 lobsters tails	160 calories
1 cup of asparagus	32 calories
1 cup of steamed carrots	53 calories
1 breadstick	12 calories
1 kiwi	42 calories

Day 18

As we aspire to make it through the rough times in life, our determination and will can be tested. During these times, remember that there can be no victory without a challenge. There's nothing you can't accomplish.

BREAKFAST

1 cup of black coffee or tea	1 calorie
1 grapefruit	37 calories
1 slice of wheat bread	78 calories

LUNCH

3.5 ounces of lean chicken breast	140 calories
1 cup of chicory greens	25 calories
½ cup of corn	45 calories
½ banana	52 calories

DINNER

1 pound of shrimp	200 calories
1 cup of zucchini	33 calories
½ squash	41 calories
1 breadstick	12 calories
½ cup of grapes	31 calories

Day 19

Your destiny lies in your hands. The great thing about being you is that only you get to decide who that is.

BREAKFAST

1 cup of black coffee or tea	1 calories
1 plum	30 calories

LUNCH

4 ounces of fresh salmon	236 calories
2 cups of spinach	24 calories
½ cup of carrots	26 calories
1 breadstick	12 calories
½ cup of strawberries	23 calories

DINNER

3.5 ounces of lean lamb chops	250 calories
1 cup of kale	42 calories
½ cup of squash	41 calories
1 Melba toast	12 calories
½ cup of raspberries	51 calories

Day 20

Believe in yourself, be confident and have faith in your inherited powers and natural abilities to achieve anything that you put your mind to.

BREAKFAST

1 cup of black coffee or tea	1 calorie
1 tangerine	47 calories
½ bagel	122 calories

LUNCH

1 pound of shrimp	200 calories
1 cup of green cabbage	25 calories
½ cup of boiled potatoes	81 calories
½ cup of blueberries	41 calories

DINNER

3.5 ounces of lean turkey breast	140 calories
2 cups of spinach	24 calories
½ cup of carrots	26 calories
1 breadstick	12 calories
½ cup of grapes	31 calories

Day 21

Positive thoughts lead to positive actions. Like a river, keep your thoughts pure and flowing. The key to your success is your determination to make it to the finish line.

BREAKFAST

1 cup of black coffee or tea	1 calorie
2 breadsticks	24 calories
1 plum	30 calories

LUNCH

3.5 ounces of lean veal	200 calories
1 cup of broccoli	50 calories
½ cup of squash	41 calories
1 breadstick	12 calories
1 peach	59 calories

DINNER

1 pound of shrimp	200 calories
1 cup of asparagus	32 calories
1 cup of tomatoes	35 calories
1 breadstick	12 calories
1 pear	51 calories

Day 22

You are just one week away from achieving your ultimate goal. Listen to the voice within and push forward. It's crunch time. You don't need anyone's permission to succeed. Believe in yourself, a confident person can't lose.

BREAKFAST

1 cup of black coffee or tea	1 calorie
½ cup of blueberries	50 calories
1 breadstick	12 calories

LUNCH

4 ounces of fresh salmon	236 calories
1 cup of romaine lettuce	30 calories
1 cup of cucumbers	14 calories
½ slice of wheat bread	39 calories
1 peach	59 calories

DINNER

4 ounces of lean turkey chops	140 calories
2 cup of collard greens	24 calories
1 cup of carrots	53 calories
1 breadstick	12 calories
1 cup of watermelon	77 calories

Day 23

It's never too late to be who you want to be. Every moment is an opportunity to recreate yourself. That is why we call it the present, these moments are gifts from God. Use them as intended and fulfill your true purpose.

BREAKFAST

1 cup of black coffee or tea	1 calorie
½ cup of strawberries	23 calories
1 breadstick	12 calories

LUNCH

3.5 ounces of lean beef	200 calories
1 cup of snow peas	26 calories
1 cup of mushrooms	21 calories
½ of white potatoes	81 calories
½ slice of wheat bread	39 calories
1 plum	30 calories

DINNER

3.5 ounces of filleted fish	160 calories
2 cups of broccoli	100 calories
1 breadstick	12 calories
1 pear	51 calories

Day 24

There is nothing you can't accomplish when you put your mind to it. Keep that mental picture of the new you in your thoughts at all times.

BREAKFAST

1 cup of black coffee or tea	1 calorie
½ of an apple	48 calories
1 Melba toast	12 calories

LUNCH

3.5 ounces of lean veal	200 calories
1 cup of romaine lettuce	30 calories
1 cup of tomatoes	35 calories
1 cup of carrots	53 calories
½ cup of blueberries	41 calories

DINNER

3.5 ounces of lean turkey breast	140 calories
1 cup of string beans	44 calories
½ cup of white potatoes	81 calories
1 breadstick	12 calories
1 pear	51 calories

Day 25

All goals are attainable. You have the power to overcome all obstacles. Let your positive thoughts lead the way to victory. As Joe Batten once said, "Doubt your doubts".

BREAKFAST

1 cup of black coffee or tea	1 calorie
1 nectarine	59 calories

LUNCH

1 pound of crab legs	200 calories
1 cup of red cabbage	20 calories
1 cup of zucchini	33 calories
1 Melba toast	12 calories
½ cup of Blueberries	41 calories

DINNER

3.5 ounces of lean beef	200 calories
1 cup of broccoli	50 calories
½ cup of white potatoes	81 calories
½ cup of strawberries	51 calories

Day 26

No one can be a better you than you. You are a magnificent being that is cable of more than you know. Take some time to go within and remember who you are. The real hero is "You".

BREAKFAST

1 cup of black coffee or tea	1 calorie
1 plum	30 calories
½ bagel	122 calories

LUNCH

1 pound of shrimp	200 calories
1 cup of romaine lettuce	30 calories
½ cup of tomatoes	17 calories
½ cup of squash	41 calories
1 Melba toast	12 calories
½ cup of honeydew	24 calories

DINNER

3.5 ounces of lean chicken breast	140 calories
1 cup of eggplant	20 calories
½ cup of Swiss chard	3 calories
2 breadsticks	24 calories
1 cup of watermelon	85 calories

Day 27

Good morning star! Today, remember that with every win there is a winner. It is your time to shine. The finish line is just around the corner.

BREAKFAST

1 cup of black coffee or tea	1 calorie
½ banana	52 calories
½ bagel	122 calories

LUNCH

1 pound of crab legs	200 calories
1 cup of green cabbage	25 calories
1 cup of cucumbers	14 calories
½ slice of wheat bread	39 calories
½ cup of blueberries	41 calories

DINNER

4 ounces of lean turkey chops	120 calories
1 cup of asparagus	32 calories
1 cup of steamed carrots	53 calories
1 breadstick	12 calories
1 kiwi	42 calories

Day 28

Think only of the results as you push forward through another day of victory. We don't make mistakes, we make choices. Chose to stay focused on the path to a new you.

BREAKFAST

1 cup of black coffee or tea	1 calorie
½ bagel	122 calories

LUNCH

3.5 ounces of filleted fish	160 calories
1 cup of broccoli	50 calories
1 cup of tomatoes	35 calories
1 Melba toast	12 calories
1 apple	81 calories

DINNER

3 ounces of lean lamb chops	250 calories
1 cup of collard greens	44 calories
1 cup of carrots	53 calories
1 tangerine	47 calories

Day 29

Take the time to appreciate the perfection in you. Even the things that you consider flaws are perfect in the eyes of God. Give yourself praise today for being his image and likeness.

BREAKFAST

1 cup of black coffee or tea	1 calorie
½ bagel	122 calories

LUNCH

2 lobsters tails	160 calories
1 cup of asparagus	32 calories
1 cup of carrots	53 calories
1 plum	30 calories

DINNER

3.5 ounces of lean veal	200 calories
2 cups of spinach	48 calories
1 cup of mushrooms	21 calories
1 cup of watermelon	77 calories

Day 30

You are the creator of your destiny, the master of your being, the gate keeper of your soul and you are always in control of you.

BREAKFAST

1 cup of black coffee or tea	1 calorie
½ cup of strawberries	23 calories
½ bagel	122 calories

LUNCH

4 ounces of scallop's	128 calories
1 cup of string beans	44 calories
½ cup of white potatoes	81 calories
1 plum	30 calories

DINNER

3.5 ounces of lean beef	200 calories
1 cup of broccoli	50 calories
1 cup of beets	8 calories
1 breadstick	12 calories
1 pear	51 calories

Part Four
CONGRADULATIONS!

You did it! You've completed "My Skinny Lil Diet". You should be feeling lighter, brighter, happier and good about yourself.

Please note that "My Skinny Lil Diet" is only recommended for thirty days. You should now increase your daily calorie intake by doubling up on the meal portions and add fitness and exercise to your daily regime to keep the weight off.

Wishing you the best on your journey through life with hopes of success and happiness.

GLOSSARY

My Skinny Lil Diet Glossary

When in doubt, remember this…If it's not in the glossary, you can't have it. Unless of course it pertains to fresh meats, vegetables and fruits that may have been missed.

Condiments:
1. Sugar substitute (coffee and tea)
2. Salt
3. Pepper
4. Fresh onions
5. Fresh garlic
6. Parsley
7. Oregano
8. Fresh squeezed lemon
9. Olive oil-1 teaspoon per meal

Other:
1. Breadsticks
2. Melba Toast

MEATS, POULTRY & FISH
*Bake, steam or broil.

Lean beef   3.5 ounce   175-200 calories
Lean veal   3.5 ounces   175-200 calories
Lean lamb chops   3 ounces   250 calories

Lean chicken breast   3.5 ounces 140-150 calories
Lean turkey breast   3.5 ounces 140- 150 calories
Lean turkey chops   4 ounces   120 calories

Fresh filleted fish 3.5 ounces   70-80 calories
Fresh scallops   4 ounces   128-130 calories
Fresh salmon   4 ounces   236-240 calories
Lobster tail   70-80 calories
Crab legs   1 pound   200 calories
Shrimp   1 pound   200 calories

VEGETABLES

&
CALORIES

*Steam, broil or eat fresh.

Bok Choy	20	Mustard greens	15
Celery	20	Chicory greens	42
Radishes	15		
Cabbage	20		
Mushrooms	21		
Cucumbers	14		
Avocado	234		
Asparagus	32		
Snow Peas	26		
Zucchini	33		
Squash	82		
Beets	8		
Carrots	53		
Broccoli	50		
Cauliflower	146		
String beans	44		
Collard greens	12		
Romaine lettuce	30		
Tomatoes	35		
Spinach	24		
Kale	42		
Okra	33		
Corn ½ cup	45		
Potatoes ½	81		
Eggplant	20		

FRUITS
&
CALORIES

Apple	95	
Banana	104	
Pear	51	
Peach	59	
Nectarine	59	
Kiwi	42	
Plum	30	
Orange	65	
Blueberries		85
Strawberries		46
Raspberries		65
Watermelon		85
Grapefruit		37
Cantaloupe		186
Cherries		75
Honeydew		48
Tangerine		47
Pomegranate		72
Cup of grapes		62

My Skinny Lil Work-Out DVD COMING 2014

I will be following up with a quick work-out video that will keep the weight off after completing 'My Skinny Lil Diet"

"My Skinny Lil Work-Out Dvd"
Will be released Spring of 2014, exclusively on Amazon.com.

Loaded with tons of fun work out routines that you can do at home right in your own living room.